Breaking the Chains

A Guide to Bariatric Surgery

By

Suzette Munson and Jennifer DeMoss

Table of Contents

Introduction

Deciding to have bariatric surgery can be an intimidating task. There are so many aspects from finding a doctor to dealing with insurance that, quite frankly, many people just become overwhelmed. We have found with our own experiences that sometimes you have so many questions you just don't know where to turn.

We developed this guide in the hopes that it will help walk you through the steps of undergoing weight loss surgery from the day you make the decision up until you get home from the hospital and beyond, including some wonderful recipes for batch-cooking that you can freeze for later!

It is our prayer that you are able to use this guide for your benefit, and that we've helped ease you into one of the biggest decisions you'll ever make in your life.

Don't forget that all of our recipes, our cooking videos, and much more can also be found on our website www.7BitesShow.com. In addition, you can find us on Facebook at www.facebook.com/7Bites and in our group www.facebook.com/groups/7Bites. Help is always at your fingertips with 7Bites on your side. Thanks for reading! Come see what we're up to!

Love and Blessings,

Suzette Munson and Jennifer DeMoss

Pre-Surgery: Everything You Need to Know

Choosing a Surgery

Choosing a surgery that's right for you can be a daunting experience. You read all the horror stories from others about different surgery experiences, and no one wants to undergo any of the negative effects from any surgery. And in doing your research, you find so much information from so many sources that you don't know who to listen to or what to think about any of them. Here, we've compiled a list of surgeries and included their risks and benefits so that you don't have to take on the nerve-wracking task on your own. There are many surgeries out there with differing risks and benefits, so there is certain to be on that will fit everyone's needs.

Gastric Bypass (Roux en Y Bypass)

This is a procedure done laparoscopically and involves a two-stage process – first, a small pouch is created using staples at the bottom of the esophagus from the top part of the stomach. The remainder of the stomach is then separated from the pouch. The pouch is connected to the middle section of the small intestine, bypassing the remaining stomach and the upper portion of the small intestine.

The bypass is among the first bariatric surgeries ever performed and has a long record of success with the first known modern version of the surgery being performed in 1967. It is also among the most successful of all bariatric surgeries with a success rate of over 90% in losing over 80% of one's excess weight.

One of the significant factors of the bypass is the "dumping syndrome" that many patients experience when they eat something they're not supposed to. For some people, this is a benefit – keeping them focused on eating the right things. For others, this is a deterrent to having the surgery.

The benefits of this surgery include a larger amount of significant weight loss along with a greater percentage of patients that keep the weight off.

The risks of this surgery include possible blood clots, malnutrition, kidney stones, gall stones, anemia, food intolerances, constipation, ulcers, osteoporosis, and possible "mushrooming" or "ballooning" of a pouch that is misused. These risks are all possibly avoidable by following surgeons' instructions and getting enough water, vitamins, and exercise.

Duodenal Switch

This is a procedure done laparoscopically and involves a two-stage process. First, a partial gastrectomy is performed, removing up to 70% of the stomach. Then the intestines are divided into two separate pathways, one that carries food and one that carries the digestive juices. The two are then brought together again in the common limb portion of the intestine. This is a malabsorptive procedure that causes a reduction in caloric absorption.

This surgery is one of the more risky of all bariatric surgeries because of the steps involved and the common length of the surgery (two stages with the second stage being over two hours in some cases). Additionally, the surgery was never developed for weight loss – rather it was created with the purpose of bile gastritis treatments. That being said, it was found that patients undergoing this procedure also experienced significant weight loss and additional health benefits after.

The success rate of the duodenal switch is one of the highest with an 80% rate – meaning that people generally lose up to 80% of their excess weight and keep it off.

The benefits of the duodenal switch include rapid weight loss with less risk for dumping syndrome than the bypass surgery, no risk of a pouch ballooning or mushrooming, large amount of weight loss and greater percentage of patients keeping the weight off.

The risks of the duodenal switch include blood loss and possible transfusion, leakage of the gastrectomy site, blood clots, malnutrition, food intolerances, constipation, kidney and/or gall stones, anemia, and ulcers. The majority of these problems can be avoided by following surgeons' orders after surgery.

Gastric Band

Also known as the Lap-Band or Realize Band, the gastric band is a procedure done laparoscopically in which a silicone band is placed around the top part of the stomach creating a pouch with a small opening in the bottom for food to pass through. On the inner portion of the band is a balloon or series of balloons around the circumference that can be filled with saline solution to cause restriction, giving a sensation of fullness after consuming up to a half cup of food.

This surgery is one with some of the fewest risks since there is no re-routing of the intestines and no portion of the stomach is removed. The entirety of the gastrointestinal system is left intact. This can be considered a great benefit to many patients. Additionally, the surgery is completely reversible whereas the bypass, duodenal switch, and vertical sleeve surgeries are not. The surgery was created in the late 1970's and was improved upon in the 1980's to the band we know now. In the 1990's, the gastric band procedure became the gastric procedure of choice for many patients and surgeons. The success rate, however, is lower than some at a 50-60% loss of excess weight. The gastric band also has the highest rate of revision surgeries done for causes including complications and failure to lose weight.

The benefits of the gastric band are that the surgery is completely reversible, the gastrointestinal system is left intact, and the band itself is customizable meaning the patient can have more or less saline in the band to make the restriction exactly what the patient needs for his or her weight loss goals.

Some of the risks involve band slippage, esophagus damage, mushrooming or ballooning of the pouch above the band, twisting of the port, hiatal hernia, gastritis, constipation, and damage from food becoming stuck in the opening around the band into the stomach.

Vertical Sleeve Gastrectomy

The vertical sleeve gastrectomy is a procedure done laparoscopically in which a significant amount of the stomach is removed. This procedure often removes part of the hunger gland in the stomach as well, reducing the feeling of hunger.

This surgery is done for people with a BMI of 35-50 and is considered one of the most common surgeries performed today. Unlike the bypass or duodenal switch, weight loss with the sleeve is significantly slower in some cases. Additionally, unlike other procedures, the stomach will return to a size and shape that will be able to hold up to a cup of food at a time, whereas with other procedures the stomach pouch will not expand with regular, proper diet and treatment. This can be considered an asset to some, and a hindrance to others, depending on what one desires out of their weight loss.

The success rate with the Vertical Sleeve is around 90% with patients losing and maintaining a loss of 60% of their excess weight or greater over a course of a couple of years. As of now there is no long term study of over 5 years on the sleeve because it wasn't until the last few years that it became a stand-alone weight loss procedure. Before then, it was used only as the first stage of the duodenal switch. When doctors discovered that patients who had the sleeve were waiting on the second portion of their surgery and losing significant weight not needing the second portion (the intestinal procedure), it began being used more frequently, and is now the most common weight loss procedure performed.

The sleeve was once thought to prevent dumping syndrome similar to what the gastric bypass patients experience, but studies now show that VSG patients can, in fact, experience dumping syndrome when consuming high sugar or high fat foods. The vertical sleeve is also not a reversible surgery.

The benefits of the sleeve are significant loss in the first six months after surgery, slower weight loss after the first six months, resulting in less chances of loose skin issues, reduced hunger, no chance of a pouch ballooning or mushrooming, and an opportunity to have a more regular "normal" diet after a period of time.

The risks of the vertical sleeve are possible leaks around the gastrectomy line, blood clots, reflux, gastritis, constipation, food intolerances, malnutrition, and dehydration. With proper care and following surgeons' orders, the majority of these issues can be avoided.

Choosing Your Surgeon and Center of Excellence

Well, now that you know what surgery you want, what about choosing the surgeon you want to perform it? Choosing the surgeon that's right for you can be as difficult as trying to choose your surgery. But it doesn't have to be. Knowing what you want out of your surgery and your doctor are assets to your health. Above all, always remember that your doctor works for you, not the other way around. It's important to keep that in mind when talking with different surgeons about different procedures.

First and foremost, if you have your heart set on a certain procedure, make sure that you find a surgeon that actually performs that procedure! You wouldn't go to a doctor that specializes in gastric banding for a RnY, and you wouldn't see a doctor that does primarily sleeve gastrectomies for a duodenal switch. Although many doctors do multiple procedures, most specialize in one particular for most surgeries. Be sure you are finding the best of the best for your area and your price point. You want to look for a surgeon that has performed many surgeries, but not so many that it seems almost unrealistic. Some doctors apply what we term a "cattle call" routine, where they do thousands of surgeries a year, focusing on the procedure rather than the patient.

With that in mind, most doctors will be able to walk you through your procedure options. If you find a good surgeon that does multiple procedures, he or she may discuss other options available to you besides the procedure you originally decided on. Don't be afraid to change your mind if it suits you, but don't feel pressured or bullied into going through with a procedure you're uncomfortable with. If you begin to feel pressured, move on to the next doctor. Even though you may be excited and anxious to get your new healthy life underway, it's important to have a doctor that will listen to and support your needs as the patients – and as the consumer!

Keep in mind that it's possible your surgery choice may change after talking to your doctor. That's what happened in Jennifer's situation:

> "I was dead set on having the lap-band surgery," she says. "I was sold on the fact that it was completely reversible and had what I thought was the least amount of risks associated with it. After talking to my surgeon, however, I changed my mind. Listening to his recommendation, I

realized the vertical sleeve fit what I was looking for and my lifestyle a whole lot better than the band did."

Be sure also that you are choosing a surgeon that fits your emotional needs as well. If you want a doctor that is more abrupt and factual, you wouldn't like to have one that is more soft-spoken and gentle natured. If, however, you prefer a gentle nature and soft voice, you wouldn't want your surgeon to be in-your-face. Make sure you and your surgeon see eye to eye on most things involving your health and your procedure. It makes for a more pleasant experience before, during, and after your surgery.

Getting Insurance Approval

Many people think that insurance won't approve your bariatric surgery for one reason or another. Most insurance companies actually WILL with the proper steps taken, even if they say they don't.

If your insurance says they don't approve surgery, talk with your doctor or bariatric surgeon. More often than not, they can walk you through approval procedure and you might find that your insurance actually DOES approve it with the proper documentation. If you're still unsure, most surgeons do have procedures to follow to ensure approval.

Many insurances also have a procedure they go through before approving surgery. Some will need documentation of a year's, or more, worth of doctors' visits for weight loss or a documented attempt of a year or more on a doctor prescribed weight loss plan. For most of us, this is easier than you might think considering we have all been obese for most of our adult lives. For most insurance purposes, just having documentation of visits where your weight was recorded will do. Check with your doctor or surgeon on this aspect and they will tell you exactly what you need to do for this to ensure approval.

Most insurances will require you undergo a psychiatric evaluation. This is not as painful or worrisome as it may seem. The purpose here is to ensure that you are mentally and emotionally prepared for the mental side of bariatric surgery. It is, after all, a huge commitment on your part. Be sure to be completely honest with the doctor you visit with about any concerns or uncertainties you might have. Not only are they there to evaluate you, but they are also there to help talk you through things you might not be comfortable with. By the time you leave the psychologists office, you should be feeling confident and uplifted about your upcoming surgery!

Suzette remembers her experience in the psychologist's office:

> "There were about 25 questions on the psychologist's list and a list of diets I had participated in through the years. I remember writing in about 20 more than what she had listed. When we spoke and reviewed the list she was shocked that I had dieted so much. My list had about 46 diet programs listed. She was relatively new to speaking with bariatric candidates and said that they had only listed the main diet programs that the

insurance companies had required. I remember telling her that I had been on a diet since I was 10 years old recovering from Rheumatic Fever when the Doctor put me on amphetamines to help me lose the weight quickly.

I would be on the diet pills for 6 weeks then off for 6 weeks until the weight was gone. Now we know that was not the best way for anyone to lose weight but back in the '60's it was an accepted treatment."

BMI requirements are generally the same across the board including a BMI of 40 or above or a BMI of 35 with co-morbidities (health issues related to your weight such as high blood pressure, high cholesterol, sleep apnea, joint pain, etc.). Some, however, are lowering their BMI requirements to under 35 with other certain requirements met.

Getting Ready for Your Surgery

After approval, a myriad of emotions will flow through you. You will experience everything from excitement and elation to anxiety and worry. All of these emotions are completely normal and okay to be feeling! It's important to remember, however, that this is the time to start preparing for your life after surgery. There are certain things that can to be done to ensure your recovery is easy and uneventful.

Go Shopping!

There are many tools of the trade that are going to make your life much easier during the first few months after surgery. We've compiled a list for you of utensils and tools that you can look for now to have on hand for later! These will help you retrain both your brain and your mouth on how to eat. Bariatric patients simply eat differently than those that haven't had surgery.

Personal Blender – there are several on the market. Look for one that has smaller cup sizes (1/2-1 cup sizes) in addition to the larger 2 cup sized containers. It's also good to look for one that has multiple blades – this will come in handy during the later eating phases of the bariatric diet.

Measuring cups – you will need both dry and liquid measures. Look for ones that go all the way down to 1/8 cup measure! This will be very helpful during the earlier stages when you're not eating as much as you will later.

Measuring spoons – you will be eating tablespoonsful of many, many things. Having a good set of spoons to use for this purpose is going be extremely helpful.

½ C portion freezer containers – these will be very helpful in storing batch cooked foods such as soups and stews for later.

Kitchen scale – this is especially helpful later on when you need to measure protein in ounces.

Water cups with oz. marked on the sides – these will help you keep track of your water intake.

Ice cube and/or ice-pop trays – especially wonderful during the hot summer months for making sugar free juice pops and/or protein pops.

Small tapas or appetizer sized plates – you can find these almost anywhere, but our favorites are found at kitchen supply stores.

Condiment bowls – these are wonderful for eating soup and stews out of – most only hold about ¼ - ½ c of food at a time.

Small tapas or appetizer sized cutlery – this can be tricky to find, but can be found in most kitchen supply stores (ask for tapas forks or appetizer spoons!). If you can't find these, baby spoons and toddler cutlery also works really well!

Mini-muffin tin – these work wonders for making everything from mini meatloaves to low-carb/high protein muffins! I suggest buying two!

Find Samples

One of the things you will need a lot of in the coming weeks is protein supplement drinks. We've found that often we'll find a brand we love before surgery, then find that after surgery we just can't tolerate them. With that in mind, it's a good idea to look up websites for different bariatric products including protein supplement drinks and find out who gives samples. Stock up on these now so you can try them after surgery. Once you find one you like and can tolerate after surgery, go ahead and order it then. That way you're not stuck wasting money on a large amount of a product you can't consume. Many nutrition stores also have samples available at low or no cost. Some web sites will even send you samples for free. It's a good idea to do your research and homework on that now. If you're having trouble finding a site or a location that offers samples, contact your surgeon – they'll be sure to have a good list of places for you and may even have some samples available in their office. You can also find samples of vitamin supplements this way as well!

Grocery Prep

It's a good idea to stock up on things that you already know you're going to need a lot of in the first week or so. For example, you might stock up on a few cases of small water bottles (8 oz.), drink mixes and drops, broths, soups, etc. As previously stated, avoid stocking up on protein drinks until after your surgery, when you know which ones to you can tolerate and which ones are more difficult for you.

Batch Cooking

This is something that many people don't think about before surgery. After surgery, there are many obstacles to us that can prevent us from getting up and making a home cooked meal. We may be tired and sore after our surgeries, and frankly our energy levels aren't going to be as high as they were prior to surgery. One of the things you can do to help yourself during this time is to have premade soups and stews in ½ c portion sizes ready for you in the freezer. That way, you can take out a container and heat it up in the microwave rather than having to sit over a stove waiting for something to cook.

Batch cooking is a very simple technique. All you do is this:

Step 1: Cook up your favorite batch of soup, stew, or similar. Make sure you are within guidelines for a bariatric diet (high protein, low carb, sugar free). If desired, you may go ahead and puree the recipe now so you don't have to do it later.

Step 2: Divide the dish into ½ c portions either in freezer containers or freezer bags. (if using the containers, do NOT fill them all the way to the top! Leave about ¼ in room in the container for expansion.

Step 3: Refrigerate for a couple of hours.

Step 4: Freeze for up to 6 months.

Step 5: When you're ready to reheat the dish, put it into the microwave at 50% power for 3 minutes. Stir. Return to microwave and heat on high for another 1-3 minutes, stirring every minute until heated through.

There are many great recipes that lend themselves well to batch cooking. Of course soups and stews are the most common, but there are other side dishes that also work well including vegetable purees and sauces. We've provided recipes for this, and other techniques in the last chapter of this book

So, now you're ready for surgery! In the next chapter, we'll discuss your surgery date and what will happen in the days following surgery.

Surgery: Before, During, and After

The day of your surgery has finally arrived! After months of waiting and anticipating it's here. Now is the time to get excited because your new life is right around the corner!

While every doctor and surgery center is different, there are a few commonalities between most of them. Here, we will discuss what you can most likely expect during your hospital stay.

Pre-Op

Before your surgery, you will meet with your doctor for some pre-op instructions. These will include your pre-op eating plan or diet, instructions on what to do the day before surgery, and how to pre-register for your surgery day. Additionally, you might receive samples of vitamins, protein powders, and other "goodies" to try out before your surgery date.

You doctor will also likely provide you with a breathing apparatus called a spirometer to practice with before surgery. You will use it to breathe in deeply and breathe out deeply. The purpose of this is to help you take deeper breaths after surgery to avoid pneumonia and other lung issues.

The Pre-Surgery Diet

Different doctors use different diets before surgery. These can range to anything from a low-carb, low-calorie eating plan to a full-blown clear liquid diet. It's important to follow your surgeon's instructions as close as possible during this time. The pre-surgery diet is designed to shrink your liver so that your doctor can access your stomach easier for surgery. An added bonus is that most pre-surgery diets are high-protein, so your body will be strengthened for healing after surgery.

In The Hospital

You will likely arrive at the hospital early in the morning. Be sure that when you get there you have your ID and any paperwork you need already filled out and ready to go. This will make admission much smoother and faster. Be prepared, after admission, you may have to wait for a bit before you are taken into the prep area.

After the admissions process, you will be taken to the OR prep room. This is where you will change into your hospital gown, you will have your vitals checked and be fitted with your IV. In some cases, you might receive special care. In Jennifer's case, for example, the nurse came in with bright yellow fuzzy socks with treading on them in the pattern of a smiley face. "I still have these socks to this day," Jennifer says. "I can't look at them and not smile." After all of these things are taken care of, the anesthesiologist will come in to administer the general anesthesia. This may be different depending on your hospital or anesthesiologist. In our case, it was a two-step process. We were given a shot in our IV, then later a mask with the anesthesia gas. You may also be given a breathing tube and catheter.

Surgical Procedure

The length of time that your procedure will take may vary depending on the type of surgery and the surgeon. Most procedures last close to an hour or so and no more than two.

During the procedure, your surgeon may periodically have a nurse or other helper come to inform whoever accompanied you how your surgery is going. This is to keep them calm and to assure them that everything is going alright.

Your doctor also might bring in a picture or video of your surgery. Jennifer still has the picture from hers. It can be either fascinating or unnerving to see these, so if you are squeamish about that kind of thing you can certainly opt out!

After Your Surgery

Waking up from anesthesia can often be a scary moment. For some, it feels as though they're choking or can't breathe. Others may feel very lightheaded and dizzy. And some experience numbness in their extremities. In any case, you will most likely feel groggy and want to sleep for a while. This is normal, and sleeping is a good and important part of healing. Jennifer's experience waking from anesthesia was not a pleasant memory for her:

> "I thought I was dying!" She recalls. "I seriously thought I was suffocating to death. I woke up and couldn't breathe at all. I started panicking and trying to scream. I think I terrified the nurse, to be honest," she chuckles. "But it was all fine.

I was completely fine. I'd had a breathing
tube in during the surgery, and my lungs
were trying to get used to breathing on
their own again. The nurse took great
care of me and was very sweet in calming
me down!"

The first few hours after surgery you will likely be sleeping a lot.
That is the anesthesia wearing off and is okay. Sleeping helps
with the healing. That being said, after the first hour or so, you
will be expected to get up and try to walk around. This is equally
important as it prevents blood clots from forming. This
condition, called thrombosis, can be life-threatening as the clots
can travel to your lungs. You might not want to, but doing this is
very important. You will be expected to do this often – at least
once an hour.

You may have leg wraps around your calves massaging them to
help prevent blood clots. It will resemble a heating pad and will
wrap around your legs like one. It's a very pleasant experience,
not painful at all, and can even be quite relaxing!

After the first few hours, you will have some tests performed to
make sure your surgery went well. You might have a sonogram
or barium test to check any staple lines or for leaks in the case
of the duodenal switch or vertical sleeve. You might have a
wound drain placed on your body as well to keep fluid buildup
from occurring around the surgical site. In some cases, you may
have tubes and/or catheters from the stomach to keep fluid out
of the stomach for a few days.

Depending on your surgery, you will have your first meal within
24-48 hours. This meal will consist of clear liquids and may
include broth, tea, sugar-free gelatin, and/or juice. You will

probably not be able to consume all of it, and that is okay. Equally okay is if you eat it all!

After your first meal, it will just be a matter of time before you are allowed to leave. Most of the time you are released as soon as you are able to eat and not become nauseous, all tests come back looking fine, and you have passed gas (this shows that your new gastrointestinal system is working properly!).

Special Cases (Out-Of-Towners)

Many patients opt to go to Mexico or even Canada for their surgeries for one reason or another. The above applies to them as well, but in many cases you might be sent to a hotel or recovery center to recover for a longer time frame. This is because the doctor wants to ensure safety during travel. These areas are often more like spas or resorts than hospitals, and it can be quite the relaxing and enjoyable experience! Take the time to relish and enjoy your stay and allow the hospital and staff to care for you properly. Be sure before your surgery, you contact a surgeon in your area that will take you as a patient for follow-up appointments and that you find a local support group to attend.

Going Home

You will likely go home after a stay of 1-3 days in the hospital. This is where the recovery process begins to get challenging. You will need to follow your surgeon's orders exactly – this will ensure you don't have any future issues with your surgery.

The first few days at home there are a few guidelines that are VERY IMPORTANT:

1) **Walk, walk, walk** – walking is super important – remember the blood clots we talked about in the above section? This is why you need to walk – it will prevent those blood clots from forming. This will also help move the gas out of your body. When you have a laparoscopic procedure done, your body cavity is often filled with gas to expand the space and make it easier for your surgeon to get to your stomach. Sometimes the gas can move and settle in other places in your body like your hips or shoulders. Walking helps move this gas out of your body.

2) **Sip, sip, sip**. Water is KEY. First of all, it will keep you hydrated. That is a very important thing at this stage. Dehydration can cause so many issues in the beginning and it's hard to get the water in. Some ways to keep sipping are to keep a water bottle or sippy cup in your hand or at your side at all times. Sip at 5, 10, or 15 minute intervals. All you need is 1-3 sips at a time to start. You will be able to drink more at a time later. We used the smaller 8oz bottles of water you can find in cases at your grocery store. These were the most convenient and the least intimidating for us. You can also add flavor to your water using drink mixes or flavor drops if you like.

3) **Rest, rest, rest**. Between the walking and the sipping you are going to want to REST! You will be up and around soon enough – now is the time for healing so be sure you are getting enough sleep. If you have a hard time sleeping because of pain or irritation, try using an incline. Other ways to ensure you're getting enough rest: NO caffeine, herbal tea before bed, sleep in

a darkened room, have some quiet time, sleep when you're sleepy.

The Second Week

The second week is a little easier than the first week. There's not quite as much pain, and you're not still groggy from the pain medicines and anesthesia. This week you will still want to walk and drink as you have been, but now it's important to begin really focusing on your eating and making sure you are getting your protein in.

This week your emotions may begin reeling. You might be thinking, "what did I do??" and start mourning your long lost friend. But just know that no amount of Funyuns and Mountain Dew can do for you what the procedure you just underwent can. Those things are temporary moments of joy that will quickly turn to anguish – especially at this stage! Trust that you did the right thing. Soon, you will start to see and feel amazing changes in your body. You will get to do things you never got to do before, you be able to feel ways you never imagined possible. As your body shrinks and changes, so will your confidence level!

It's important to point out how important protein is at this stage. We all fall into the trap of "is protein really THAT important?" as we seek out other alternative foods. YES, protein really is THAT important! First of all, it helps with the healing process. Protein is important for rebuilding muscle and flesh – that's exactly what's going on in your body right now as your staple lines and sutures are healing. Protein is a key component in that. Also, your body needs substance to keep going. While veggies and carbs can give you a small burst of energy, energy from protein lasts longer and keeps your blood sugar more regulated.

It might also be a good idea to start a VERY low-impact exercise routine – WALKING! You've been doing it already on a daily basis to keep blood clots at bay. Now it's time to do it for activity! You can walk a track, around the block, even just around your living room. Some people love to go walk a superstore or mall. Whatever gets you out and walking. It's important to NOT over-exert yourself however. You are still healing from major surgery, and you have likely not been released for any strenuous exercise. Take it slow and easy and don't push yourself too hard at first. If you get winded or feel any pain anywhere in your body, stop and rest. But do remember that exercise is a very important part of the recovery process!

As time goes on and your body heals more and more you will begin to notice things you never imagined. You might be able to walk up a flight of stairs without pain or being out of breath, you might be able to sit on the floor and be able to get up unassisted, you might be able to cross your legs for the first time in years. You will start to notice changes in your appearance as well. You'll find a collarbone, a waistline, and in some cases, even smaller feet! Your recovery time will likely last around 2-6 weeks. After this time, your doctor will release you for more vigorous activity. When that happens, the sky becomes the limit!

The surgery is over, you are well on your way to recovery. The new, healthy you is up to you now!

The Emotional Rollercoaster

Something you will experience is an "emotional rollercoaster" of sorts. It happens to everyone and is perfectly normal.

You will likely experience a moment or two when you're questioning your decision to undergo weight loss surgery. You may be concerned about several aspects, including how much weight you're going to lose, any complications that might occur, or even saying goodbye to your best friend – FOOD.

Know that all emotions you feel are completely normal and healthy!

Here's what your emotional rollercoaster might look like:

You might start out feeling excited – you're going to finally get the help you need to get healthy!
Next, you might feel anxious – will insurance approve you? Will you be okay during surgery? Will you have any of the complications people talk about? There are a million different concerns that may be floating through your head right now.
Next, you might feel a little sad and depressed. Some people actually undergo a mourning period. After all, you're being separated from something that was a comfort and a friend to you. For some, it's almost like a person about to undergo rehab.

It's important to say that your rollercoaster might look different. Some may have more twists and turns than the biggest roller coaster on Earth. Others might be more simplistic with only a few peaks and valleys. You might not even experience a roller coaster at all, but rather you might your time in a state of joy and elation. But it's important to be prepared and know what to do to eleviate some of the more negative feelings.

Find Support

This is key to success in any weight loss effort, but even more key in the case of bariatric surgery. If your family or close friends aren't supportive of your choice, find someone who IS. Go to a local support group, find an online forum or chat room, or find a facebook group (or other social media platform). It's important to have someone to talk to, to vent to, to cry to, to scream to, and to give you 100% support.

Journaling

Journaling can be a vital tool in success. You can say things in a journal that you can't say out loud, and often you can write out a solution to a problem without realizing it until you go back and re-read it later. Some days you might write a little, others you might write a lot – it really doesn't matter. But having that outlet can be helpful.

Counseling

For many of us, we will be recovering from the biggest, most challenging addiction on the planet. Food addiction is no joke and it's not something to be taken lightly. Finding a good addiction counselor that specializes in eating disorders and/or bariatric surgery can be a lifesaver!

Get Busy!

Find something to do that doesn't involve food! Go volunteer somewhere, find a fun hobby like dancing or bike riding, or something creative like painting or crochet. Finding something to do that will keep your mind off of your worries will be helpful both before and after surgery. Before surgery, it will keep you focused on something positive. After, it will be something to keep your mind off of food and eating. This is also a tactic used in many addiction recovery programs. They advocate art, especially, because the patient can use painting, sculpture, or writing as an outlet and express what they are going through in an outward manner without returning to the addictive substance. In our case, that would be food. Of course, it's impossible to escape food entirely, but finding something that will prevent you from focusing on it is quite helpful and healthy.

Batch Cooking Recipes

As discussed in chapter one, batch cooking certain foods prior to your surgery date is an excellent way to help your recovery go smoothly. These recipes can be done quite simply, then frozen in ½ C portion sizes for reheating later.

How To

1) **Cook your meal.** The recipes below can give you some guideline on some simple and easy recipes to make and freeze for later.

2) **Cool it completely.** Freezer burn is NOT something we want to encounter when we're tired and listless and just want a bowl of soup. Cooling you meal completely in the refrigerator helps prevent this from happening.

3) **Store in ½ C portions.** If desired, you may go ahead and puree your soup before this step! For most bariatric patients, ½ is about all we can hold at any one time. Most of the time, in the beginning, we can't even eat that much. Storing in smaller portions like this keeps us from trying to eat too much and hurting ourselves or making ourselves sick. You can use small freezer bags by placing the bag into a measuring cup and folding over the bag to prevent it from falling into the cup. Put your portion of food into the bag and seal it tightly. This process will also work with sealer machines. Alternatively, you can find freezer and/or storage containers (bowls) in small sizes that will also work well for this. Be sure you leave some room at the top of these, however, because liquids expand when they freeze. If the container is too full, it might burst once frozen.

4) **Freeze.** Store in your freezer for up to 6 months for most recipes!

5) **Reheat.** There are two ways you can reheat your portion – in the microwave or on the stove. If you are reheating it on the stove, it is helpful to slightly thaw it first by running water over the container for a few minutes. If you are reheating it in the microwave:

>1. Remove it from the storage bag, if you used one, and place in a microwave-safe container. If you used the storage container with a lid, you can skip this step, but remove the lid and place it back on the container loosely.
>
>2. Microwave at 50% power for 90 seconds. Stir. Microwave another 90 seconds on high, stirring every 30 seconds.
>
>3. Be sure to allow it to cool before eating it!

Recipes

These are just a few of the recipes we've formulated for this purpose. Be sure to check out our website and YouTube channel for more great ideas!

Chicken and Vegetable Soup

This soup is rich in protein and fiber, and is made with bone broth that is a rich, fortified stock made from the bones of the chicken.

The Bone Broth:

1 whole chicken
4 qts. Cold water
2 onions, halved
2 carrots, peeled and cut into hunks
2 ribs celery, ends removed and cut into hunks
4 cloves garlic, peeled and slightly smashed or bruised
1 bunch flat-leave (Italian) parsley
3 sprigs rosemary
2-3 bay leaves
2 T salt
1 T black pepper
2 T apple cider vinegar

1. Place chicken in a slow cooker or in a large stock pot. Cover with water (you might need more or less than the given 4 quarts listed – you will need enough to cover the chicken completely by 1 inch). Put remaining ingredients on top and put the lid on. If using the slow cooker, cook on low for up to 24 hours or on high for up to 12 hours. If doing this on the stove, bring to a boil over medium heat, reduce heat to low and simmer for up to 3 hours.

2. Remove from heat (or turn off slow cooker) and allow to cool with the lid on for up to an hour.

3. Strain broth into a large bowl or container. Discard vegetables, but keep the chicken.

4. Broth may be frozen in ice cube trays and transferred to plastic bags for later use.

The Soup:

Meat from the chicken used in the above recipe, chopped
2 qts bone broth
2 onions, chopped
2 carrots, chopped
2 ribs celery, Chopped
3 cloves garlic, peeled and smashed
1 C chopped squash (any summer or winter variety will do, depending on your taste and preference!)
Salt and pepper to taste

1. In a stock pot sautee onions, carrots, and celery until just tender. Add remaining ingredients and stir well to combine.

2. Bring to a boil over medium heat. Reduce heat, pop the lid on and cook for about 30 minutes.

3. Follow freezing directions.

Jen's Fun Chili

Okay, true story. Mom HATES my chili. That's okay. I absolutely love it and so does just about everyone else I make it for. Except my mother! This is a good one for just about everyone. If you're on full liquids or pureed foods, just run it through the food processor for a few seconds! I like to top mine with some plain Greek yogurt and a touch of cheddar cheese!

1 lb. lean ground beef or venison
1 onion, chopped
1 bell pepper, chopped
2 cloves garlic, chopped
1/4 C chili powder
1 tsp cumin
1 tsp oregano
2 tsp salt
1 tsp black pepper
2 tsp onion powder
2 tsp garlic powder
1 tsp paprika
1 tsp cinnamon
2 T brown sugar substitute
1 6 oz. can tomato paste
1 16 oz. can crushed tomatoes
cayenne pepper to taste

1. In a soup pot, brown meat with veggies in about 1 T olive or coconut oil.

2. Add seasonings and mix well.

3. Add tomato paste and cook for a minute or two.

4. Add wine (if using), tomatoes, and stock and stir.

5. Cook over medium heat for a couple of hours or transfer to slow cooker and cook on low for up to 12 hours or on high for up to 8 hours.

6. Follow freezing instructions.

Suzette's No-Roux Gumbo

This is a delicious alternative to the traditional gumbo with the high-fat and high-carb roux. This lends itself well to the batch cooking method as well, and is equally delicious pureed! This is also a good one for those that can't tolerate overly spicy foods. There is more flavor than heat, and the hot sauce can be omitted completely if needed. There are a lot of ingredients in this recipe but chopped onions, bell pepper and celery are available in the fresh food section and in the frozen food section. Using the rotisserie chicken makes this very simple because you just pull the chicken off the bone and dump it in the broth.

2 tablespoons Olive Oil
2 tablespoons butter
2 medium Onions chopped finely about 2 cups
1 cup Bell Pepper chopped finely
½ cup celery chopped finely
2 cloves garlic chopped finely
2 cups white wine

2 quarts or more of chicken broth or stock

1 lb. good smoked sausages

1 ½ cups of shredded Chicken (deli rotisserie chicken is great, canned chicken can be used but it is not as good as fresh shredded chicken. Turkey can be substituted)

1 pound of Shrimp

1pound of un breaded frozen okra (canned can be used but it is slimy so be prepared. This is the thickening agent)

2 Tablespoons Worcestershire Sauce

2-3 teaspoons of Cajun Seasoning, we use mild

1 ½ tablespoons of Hot Sauce (to your taste)

1 large can of diced tomatoes

1. In a large pot, brown the vegetables in the olive oil and butter. Cook till they are translucent.

2. Add the White Wine and the seasonings.

3. Add the smoked okra, sausage and shredded chicken.

4. Bring to a strong boil for about 15-20 minutes - check to make sure the okra is beginning to soften.

5. Turn off the heat and add the shrimp.

6. Follow freezing directions

Suzette's Beef Stew

This recipe was slightly modified from our original to take out the potatoes – most doctors want us eating the lowest carb diet possible during the first few phases!

1 to 1/12 lbs. of stew meat
1 ½ cup of carrots
1 can tomato paste
4 cups beef stock
2 sprigs of rosemary (you can chop or lay in the pot, dry rosemary use 1 teaspoon)
a few dashes of Worcestershire sauce
salt and pepper to taste

1. Salt and pepper stew meat - till you can see it (the salt and pepper, that is)!

2. Brown stew meat in a hot skillet with about 2 tablespoons of olive or vegetable oil, add oil to the pan as needed.

3. Put tomato paste, stock and vegetables into the crock pot or cooking pot

4. Add the browned meat, pour water or stock into the hot pan to deglaze and add to the pot.

5. Using a crockpot set on low for 8-10 hours. Cooking on the stovetop at a simmer until vegetables are tender.

Hot Tomato Appetizing Drink

This seems like a strange one to include, but it makes a TON and is a great evening drink or wonderful for cold weather.

3 cups of chicken broth/stock
2 cups of low-sodium tomato juice
1 Tablespoon Onion Juice
1/2 teaspoon salt or to taste
1/8 teaspoon garlic powder
1/8 teaspoon coarse pepper
1/8 teaspoon celery powder

1. Combine ingredients in a sauce pan and bring to a boil. Turn off heat.

2. Follow freezing directions

Suggestion: Pour into mini muffin tins or ice cube trays and freeze portions. Place in a freezer bag and use as needed.

Afterward

We hope that we have made the process of obtaining bariatric surgery and going through the first few days of recovery less difficult and that we've alleviated some of the anxiety you might be feeling about your decision. Remember that the decision to have weight loss surgery is a personal one and one that you and you alone should make for yourself. While there are people that look down on bariatric surgery as the "easy way out" to weight loss, it is certainly NOT easy – by any realm of the imagination. There is still a lot of hard work and dedication ahead on your part, but remember that you have a team around you ready to support you! It's worth mentioning again that you can always find recipes, blog posts, and information on our blog www.7BitesShow.com and you can also get in touch with us via Facebook and YouTube. We are always ready to give advice, lend a hand, pray with you, pray for you, and to just listen!

Please keep in touch with us and tell us about your journey!

Email us at: SevenBitesShow@gmail.com
Google + : **7 Bites**
Facebook us at: www.facebook.com/7Bites
Tweet Us: **@7BitesShow**
Pin us: **www.pinterest.com/7Bites**

Thank you for reading! Don't forget to shoot us a message to let us know how we've helped you!